GOD'S MEDICINE

By

Florastine Jethroe

DISCLAIMER

I am not a physician and in no way purport myself to be a physician or medical professional of any kind. This book does not propose to replace the service of anyone's family practitioner, or physician, that should be consulted for conditions requiring medical services. Consult a physician, holistic doctor, or health care professional before starting any herbal solution or remedy for any condition. Should a person choose to use the information disclosed in this book for self-treatment, or for treating others, the author, publisher(s), and/or distributors assume no responsibility.

TABLE OF CONTENTS

This book is lovingly dedicated to all of God's Saints, especially the late Prophet Cletus Smith who kept prophesying to me about the book.

Acknowledgements

In writing this book, I had a great deal of help, advice, encouragement, and inspiration. Special thanks to those people who said, " Maybe you should write a book about herbs," Sister Martha Chism and Brother Cletus Smith. I would also like to thank Marva Harris and my daughters, Ywanzia Ralleigh and Rene Terry, for typing, and granddaughter Danielle Williams, for editing. Sincerest thanks to Lotus Press for granting permission to use excerpts from "Back to Eden" by Jethro Kloss.

May God bless all who read this book.
Honoring God in it all.

God's Medicine
By Florastine Jethroe

FORWARD

According to my grandmother (and Jethro Kloss), there is a reason for the expression "Mother Earth". The earth is our mother, in the sense that we get our food and nutrients from her, just like a baby gets nourishment from his or her mother when nursed. Psalms 104:14 reads *"He causeth the grass to grow for the cattle and herb for the service of man..."* Herbs grow from the earth and they bring about miraculous changes in a person who needs a singular ingredient to bring him back to well being again. However, if one doesn't believe in herbal medicine and needs a diagnosis, or a prescription for a specific health problem, he or she should see a physician who can handle his or her case according to the laws of medicine. It is better to have a healthy body when trying to reach "God-Realization" than one filled with pain, anguish, and sickness.

I myself have endured the pain and strife that sickness can bring about in one's life. I was diagnosed with stage three-breast cancer in the fall of 2014 and started chemotherapy in January of the following year. I underwent 4 months of intense chemotherapy treatments, and two surgical procedures. One procedure removed all of my breast tissue, and the other was for reconstruction. I remember how tragic it was for me to see myself dismembered, with tubes hanging from my chest cavity. Yet, I did what I was advised to do by the MD's because they were the experts. They knew about all of the statistics and the "standard of care" that "typically" worked for breast cancer patients with my diagnosis. So, I adhered to another year of immunotherapy and 6 weeks of radiation to reduce the chance of reoccurrence. I completed my last treatment in April of 2016 and, after several follow-up visits, was determined to be in remission by my Practitioners.

Four months after finishing treatments I noticed pain in my left hip that began to worsen by the winter of that year. My primary care physician diagnosed me with arthritis, however, after prescribing several different medications that did not work, my oncologist referred me to a Physical Therapist who specialized in working with cancer patients. She used dry needle therapy to treat me for the pain in my hip, which worked for a time. However, by the summer of 2017 the pain had become excruciating and I was taken to the hospital for a high fever. It was there that my husband and I were informed that the pain was due to a reoccurrence of breast cancer that had metastasized to the bones in my left hip. It had also traveled to my lower back, left shoulder, lungs, and parts of my spine and chest. This time it was much worse than it was back in 2014, and it was considered terminal.

I could not believe what my ears were hearing, however having heard such terrible news before I didn't react right away; I put some thought into it. See, I was treated for Acute Lymphoblastic Leukemia (A.L.L) as a child in 1993. The first round of chemotherapy proved to be successful until I relapsed in '96. Thus, as an adult, although the news was devastating, I knew from my experience that cancer can and will sometimes return after completion of a "successful" chemotherapy regiment. This is because everybody is different. The "standard of care" does not work for everyone, and statistics do not prove that what works for umpteen thousand people will work for you. There is no "typical" human body because we are all unique.

I remembered my grandmother always had something for me to drink, or a tea that she recommended for me to cleanse my system during treatments for A.L.L. So after round 2 of intense chemo and radiation treatments for Leukemia there was no reoccurrence. Therefore, this time I chose to pass on chemotherapy and take a holistic approach to healing my body of breast cancer.

Wholesome living is so important to me because I have seen in my own life that it works. Today, I am integrating holistic eating with immunotherapy and it is working. In addition to working with an Integrative Meds MD and a Dietician, I also continue to read and learn about healthy eating. I drink herbal teas, and I've cut a lot of unhealthy foods and drinks out of my diet. I have continued to work at this, and can honestly say that today (only six months after being diagnosed with a terminal illness) the cancer in my hip is treated, I am pain free, and I am healthier than I have ever been. I persist to educate myself, exercise, and make wholesome changes to my diet because it is a life long way of living, not a temporary process. I look forward to the day where I will say that I am cancer free, but for now I can say that I am moving in that direction and it would not have been achieved without holistic a diet.

I have found this book to be helpful and informative while on my journey towards optimal health. My grandmother believes that one can concentrate better upon God, or any subjective experience in life, with a healthy mind and body; and I agree.

D.D Williams

PERSONAL EXPERIENCE

During five years of experimenting with herbs I learned things that were of value to my health. I have tried all kinds of herbs for the benefit of my family and myself. I am writing about my experience so that others may have the benefit of what I have found to be helpful.

To begin, an herb is a non-woody plant that dies into the ground after flowering. The term herb is often applied, more generally, to any plant that has been used for medicinal purposes, nutritional purposes, food seasoning, coloring, or dyeing of other substances.

My first experience with the herb involved peppermint tea. I would go to my sister in law's house and pull peppermint leaves from her backyard. I would go home, rinse them off, put them in a paper bag, let them dry, and make tea from them later. The reason this first

"Your body will talk to you and teach you if you listen and obey it."

Flo

experience is so important is because, when I reached my

forties, my doctor diagnosed me with gallstones, and he wanted to operate. I knew enough about the use of herbs to heal the body, so I bought a book about herbs and started using an herbal remedy. To treat my condition, I made a gallon of peppermint tea and drank it for a week. I drank olive oil and lemon juice and I'd lay on my right side with my hips elevated with two pillows underneath them. This caused the oil to run into **the** mouth of the gallbladder so that the gallstones could pass, and they did. I used dandelion flowers for tonic, which cleansed the blood stream. I have found that no unwanted bacteria can live in a clean blood stream.

THE BODY IS THE TEMPLE

The body is the temple of the Holy Spirit. We should like to keep it clean, body, soul, and spirit. Our bodies are like motors in a vehicle. If we don't keep the oil clean the engine and all the other parts will clog up.

Let's compare a tree with the human body. When a tree lacks the essential nutrients, it will become weak and die. The same holds true for our bodies, without the proper nutrients our bodies break down. God placed nutrients in the ground for a tree to stand tall, and so we should keep the essential nutrients in our bodies so that we can live healthy as well. I have learned that every man-made vitamin can be found in the ground. God revealed to me that man has taken from earth and created synthetic products that are weaker. This has been done in order that the condition last longer and man profit financially. Thus, a person seeking spiritual enlightenment will become acquainted with herbs, minerals, plants, and flowers for improving his or her health. Then, the person can concentrate on spiritual growth instead of being distracted with illness and pain. We may continually increase our life span, and lead healthier lives when we consider the importance of keeping our blood stream clean. The bible teaches that our blood is our life source. I use *dandelion* or *sassafras* tea, at least once a month, as a means of cleansing the blood. I use vitamins to supplement my diet when I know I am not eating a balanced meal. This process keeps me filled with energy. As a younger woman, my body essentially lacked energy due to my smoking and drinking habit. To be honest, I was sick of myself, but one day the sweet Savior our Lord Jesus came to me in a dream. He took away the taste for tobacco and alcohol from my body. He led me to people who had knowledge of herbs, and from these people, I learned how to cleanse my lungs and body of years of toxic poisoning.

"For the life of the flesh is in the blood..." Leviticus 17:11, and in the same chapter, fourteenth verse, *"For it is the life of all flesh; the blood of it is for the life thereof..."* Health and happiness depend upon the blood stream containing all sixteen elements. When one is missing, disease results in some form. To make the blood stream pure and health

producing, eat food in its natural state as much as possible. In addition, drink freely of pure water, bathe frequently, exercise in pure air and sunshine, and use non-poisonous herbs that were given for the service of man.

Psalms 104:14, *"He causeth the grass to grow for the cattle, and herb for the service of man: that he may bring forth food out of the earth."*

In order to get and maintain healthy bodies we must learn to read our bibles, have repenting spirits, eat the right foods, and keep our blood stream clean. The blood is to your body what the sap is to the plant, the building material.

"Don't take on the impossible task of ridding yourself of some bad habit or sin in your life! When you've truly had enough and you know in your heart you want to change, just go to God, through Christ Jesus. In His name, He will take it from you."

Flo

FOOD CONSUMPTION & HERBALISM

The principle abuse in eating is the consumption of excessive amounts of starch and glutinous foods. These are foods such as: white bread, cooked cereals, potatoes, pies, cakes, white flour pasta, pastries of all kinds, chocolate milk, thick soups, and gravy, just to name a few. Eating these foods in excess can form mucous and acid in the body. This does not digest well and can ferment in the digestive tract, forming alcohol and acetic acids. This can clog the mucous membranes and produce catarrh, colds, and trouble in the bowels. For thousands of years herbs have been used to correct these physical conditions.

Herbalism is the study and practice of using herbs for medicinal and therapeutic purposes. This may not be a term in your active vocabulary but it is a reality in your life. The mustard on the restaurant table and many of the spices on your kitchen shelf come from herbs. Many of the vegetables in your salads are herbs. If you have a yard, or a garden, there may be plants growing there (whether naturally or by your own design) that are herbs. Whether you are a beginner, whose concerned with herbs, or have been confined to clearing dandelions and other weeds out of your lawn, or an "old timer" whose fingers are practically rooted in your own herb garden, this book is intended to bring you pleasure and useful information.

Historically, man have used, both individually and in combination, any of the following: magic, sorcery, prayer, music, crude operations, psychotherapy, physical therapy, along with remedies prepared from plants, animals, and minerals to treat the body. Of all these, plant remedies represent the most consistent and universal form of treatment. Whatever else men may have done in the name of medicine, plants were the basic source of therapeutic products, for both professional and folk use, from the earliest days until the twentieth century. Unfortunately, plants have been burdened with a mass of both pagan and Christian superstitions that have overshadowed their wonderful properties.

The twentieth century was not kind to the old knowledge and traditions of herbalism. In the rush for faster, more efficient, more convenient ways to do things, we left old ways behind without hesitation. In the mist of it all, there were a few voices that opposed the headlong rush from nature, but with little success. Progress in our time has been based on waste. We throw away things when they have been used or made obsolete by something newer and supposedly better. Old herbal knowledge has been replaced by the latest techniques, natural remedies by synthetic drugs, natural foods by processed convenient products, plants, dyes, and coloring by chemical substitutes, common sense and self-reliance by deference to "specialist" and lack of self-confidence.

PLANTS & HERBS OF THE BIBLE

Genesis 9:20 – 21

Vine – a plant whose stem requires support and which climbs and creeps, by tendrils, along the ground or against any nearby object. There are several kinds of different *vines;* one is that of the *grapevine*. Grapes can be dried for raisins and the juice can be made into wine. Raisins contain tartaric acid, which aids in improving one's digestion. They are an excellent source of fiber, rich in iron, and when eaten regularly helps the teeth to stay strong.

Deuteronomy 8:7 – 8

Fig Tree – is very common to Palestine. It is a tree that bears edible fruit, called a *fig*. To *"sit under one's own vine and one's own fig tree"* became a proverbial expression among the Jews. It denotes peace and prosperity. For internal use, the *fig* has mild laxative properties and is often used in combination with *senna* and *carminative herbs*. The fresh *fig*, roasted and cut in half, makes a good emollient poultice for boils and small tumors. The stem and leaves contain an acrid milk juice that can be used to remove warts.

I Kings 7: 18 – 20

Pomegranate – a small tree that bears *pomegranate* fruit. The *pomegranate* fruit is a thick skinned, reddish, tart flavored berry about the size of an orange. It contains seeds in a crimson pulp. *Pomegranate* seeds have been used as a remedy for tapeworm since the time of the ancient Greeks. It is good for internal and external use; for skin problems; as a gargle for throat and mouth irritation; as a vaginal douche; and for diarrhea. Caution: large doses of the rind can cause cramps, vomiting, and other unpleasant effects. Consult a physician or holistic doctor before use.

I Kings 6:23

Olive Tree – the *olive tree* was among the most abundant and characteristic vegetation of Judea. It is a small tree that produces the *olive* fruit. In order to make oil, the fruit either was bruised in a mortar, crushed in a press loaded with wood or stones, or trodden with the feet. The Jews used oil for anointing the body after a bath, as well as giving the skin and hair a smooth comely appearance before an event. The leaves could be used for an antiseptic, astringent, and a tranquilizer.

Olive oil can be used as a cholagogue, demulcent emollient, or laxative. A decoction of the leaves on the inner bark of the tree is effective against fever. If the leaves are infused to have a tranquilizing effect, it can be helpful for nervous tension. *Olive oil*, taken internally, increases the secretion of bile and acts as a laxative by encouraging muscular contraction in the bowels. It is also soothing to mucous membrane and is said to dissolve cholesterol. *Olive oil* is also useful externally for burns, bruises, insect bites, sprains, and intense itching (pruritus). With alcohol it makes a good treatment for dandruff. One of its most common uses is a base for liniments and ointments.

Genesis 25: 29 – 34

Lentil – a leguminous plant bearing seeds that resemble small beans. These *lentil* beans were used in the sod pottage that Jacob made. *Lentils* are a good source of B vitamins, minerals, protein, and fiber. Eating *lentils* can help lower cholesterol and keep blood sugar levels low.

Isaiah 1:8

Cucumber – is a plant that is rooted from the ground with creeping vines that wrap and support the plant by tendrils. *Cucumbers* are the fruit of the plant. *Cucumbers* help to eliminate water from the body, which is beneficial for those with heart and kidney problems. It also helps to dissolve uric acid accumulations such as kidney and bladder stones. A *cucumber* salad is good for chronic constipation. *Cucumber* juice has beneficial effects on the intestines, lungs, kidneys, and skin. The juice can also be applied to bedsores, burns, and inflammation of the skin. The most effective *cucumbers* are those that are fully ripe, which is indicated by a yellow color.

Numbers 11:5

Garlic – is a bulbous flowering plant that can grow up to two feet high and produces a hermaphrodite flower. *Garlic* stimulates the digestive organs and therefore relieves various problems associated with poor digestion. When used as an expectorant, it relieves chronic stomach and intestinal catarrh, as well as chronic bronchitis. *Garlic* also regulates the liver and gallbladder. It is helpful for all intestinal infections, such as dysentery, cholera, typhoid, and paratyphoid fevers. It also helps to restore the imbalance due to putrefactive intestinal bacteria.

The tincture of the *garlic* lowers blood pressure and helps to counteract arteriosclerosis. It has beneficial effects on blood circulation and the heart, which can bring relief for many common body complaints. A cool or warm mixture of *garlic* extract and distilled water can be used as an enema for intestinal worms and other parasites. A warm enema will relax the bowels, but a cool enema can be used if the bowels are weak. Caution: consult a physician or holistic doctor before starting an enema.

Matthew 23:23

Anise – is one of the old fashioned herbaceous plants with many valuable properties. It has a flavor that would tickle the palate of most people, also known as *aniseed*, it's used to flavor candy. *Aniseed* will also prevent fermentation and gas in the stomach and bowels, as well as check griping in the bowels when taken as a hot tea. *Aniseed* is a very good remedy for nausea and colic.

Numbers 11: 7

Coriander – is an annual herb. It is a soft plant whose leaves are commonly known as cilantro. *Coriander seed* is the dry fruit of the plant, which contains a citrus flavor. The flavor of the *coriander seed* can make cookies, cakes, candies, and salads taste especially delicious. *Coriander* makes a good stomach tonic and is very strengthening for the heart. *Coriander* will allay griping caused by other laxatives and expel wind from the bowels. It is also good for flavoring other unpleasant tasting herbs.

Matthew 23:23

Cumin – is another annual herbaceous flowering plant. The plant's fruit contains a seed, which is dried and used to flavor food. *Cumin* is a key ingredient used in chili powder. It can aid in digestion, helps to relieve colic and various sorts of headaches.

Matthew 23:23

Mint – or menthe is an aromatic perennial herb. It is a flowering plant that has rendered over ten indistinct species. _Mint_ is used in desserts, green salads, teas, and other drinks. _Mint_ tea or oil can be taken for nervousness, insomnia, cramps, coughs, migraines, poor digestion, heartburn, nausea, abdominal pain, and various other problems related to anxiety.

Ruth 2:14

Vinegar – is generally a liquid made of acetic acid and water. _Apple cider vinegar_ is a type of _vinegar_ made from apple must and cider. It is very beneficial to the body and should be included in your life. The advantages from the use of _apple cider vinegar_ are many and diverse. It is a natural antiseptic and has the ability to kill bacteria in the digestive tract. It aids in digestion because it balances the digestive juices in the stomach. _Apple cider vinegar_ improves the body's metabolism. It helps to prevent toxemia, improves the blood stream, works against obesity, and heals wounds faster. About two teaspoons of _apple cider vinegar_ a day will help keep the doctor away.

Proverbs 7:17

Aloe Vera – is a succulent plant with no stem. The leaves are thick and contain a gel best known for its healing properties. *Aloe Vera* can be used for cleaning out the colon and promote menstruation. It cleans morbid matter from the stomach, liver, kidneys, spleen, and bladder. It is excellent to put over burns, radiation burns, cuts, and bruises. For those who sing or speak, *aloe vera* clears the throat.

Ezekiel 27:18 – 19

Calamus – is also known as *Sweet Flag*. It is a perennial flowering plant. *Sweet Flag* is known for its beneficial effects on the stomach. It stimulates appetite and helps to relieve acute and chronic dyspepsia, gastritis, and hyperacidity. Chewing the root is also said to relieve pyrosis or heartburn. For smokers, however, chewing the dried root tends to cause mild nausea, thus making *sweet flag* useful in breaking the smoking habit.

Revelation 18:11 – 13

Cinnamon – is a spice that comes from inside the bark of trees in the *cinnamomum* class. *Cinnamomum* is a type of evergreen tree known for its aromatic scent. Trees and shrubs from this species contain the aroma in their bark and leaves. The rind of the *laurus cinnamomum* is mentioned in Exodus 30:23 as a key ingredient in the holy anointing oil. Generally, *cinnamon* is used as a spice, however the oil from the *cinnamon* leaf has also been found to be useful in killing mosquito larvae.

Exodus 30:34 – 35

Galbanum – an aromatic gum that is secreted from the *Ferula Gummosa* plant. In this scripture it was employed in the preparation of the sacred incense. Occasionally, It is still used as an ingredient for certain perfumes.

Matthew 17:20

Mustard Seed – is the seed of *mustard plants*. It can grow anywhere from two to seven feet high. *Mustard seeds* are rich in oil and protein, and are good for seasoning salads, vegetables, dressing, marinades, as well as for pickling.

Matthew 2:11

Myrrh – is the scented resin that comes from certain trees and shrubs in eastern Africa and Arabia. Using *myrrh* as a gargle and mouthwash is good for sores in the mouth, throat, and gums. *Myrrh* helps relieve coughs due to asthma and other chest related problems. It can also be taken internally for bad breath, loose teeth, sores, and wounds.

Stacte is the product of *myrrh*. In ancient sources it is described as the extracted parts from the *myrrh* resin, or the product of *myrrh* after being heated over fire. In Exodus 30:34 it was mixed with equal parts of onycha, galbanum, and frankincense and burned as holy incense.

<u>*Ruth 2:17*</u>

Barley – is a member of the grass family. It is one of the most important of the cereal grains and the most hardy of them all. It is said to be a good source of nutrition for those with throat or stomach problems. Mixing *barley* water with milk makes a soothing preparation for stomach and intestinal problems. *Barley* has also been recommended for feverish conditions. The demulcent properties of cooked *barley* make it useful as an external application for tumors and sores.

Exodus 12:8

Yellow Dock – is a perennial flowering plant from the buckwheat family. The root of the plant is excellent and effective as a remedy for impure blood; it tones up the entire system. It helps with eruptive diseases, scrofula glandular tumors, swelling, leprosy, cancer, ulcerated eyelids, syphilis, running ears, and pruritus.

Job 30:4

Juniper – is a coniferous plant that comes in over fifty different species. *Junipers* are very abundant in the desert of Sinai and provide shade and protection, from both heat and storm, to travelers. The oil extracted from both the berry and the wood of the *juniper* has long been used as a home remedy for backache and kidney trouble. The doses are used as four to six drops on a little cube of sugar.

Psalm 51:7

Hyssop – is an herbaceous plant known for its medicinal and cleansing properties. *Hyssop* is an old Biblical remedy, David said *"Purge me with hyssop, and I shall be clean; wash me, and I shall be whiter than snow."* It is valuable for clearing quinsy due to asthma, colds, grippe, and all chest infections. Using *hyssop* loosens phlegm in the lungs and throat. For fevers, make *hyssop* tea by simmering a tablespoon of the herb in a pot of boiling water for ten minutes, and then drink a glass every hour. This will cause one to perspire, discharge the kidneys, bladder, and bowels.

It also kills body lice and helps to relieve eye trouble.

SICKNESS IN THE BIBLE & THE NATURAL REMEDY

Luke 16:20

Ulcers are a slow healing open sore in which tissue breaks down. Ulcers may form where the skin is cut or broken and does not readily heal. When the tissue has been destroyed by a burn, cut, or wound of any kind, pus may result. Ulcers can also form internally as well.

Treatment: A light diet is necessary, and the food must be well digested. The bowels should move two or three times a day. Use laxative herbs and enemas to help move the bowels. Steep one teaspoon of *golden seal* and one and a half teaspoon of *myrrh* in a pint of boiling water. Take a teaspoon of this solution six times a day. For an external ulcer, mix together one teaspoon of *powdered golden seal* and one teaspoon of *myrrh*, sprinkle it on the ulcer after it has been thoroughly washed. Cover it loosely with a bandage.

Any one of the following plants can be used externally for the treatment of ulcers as well. *Bayberry* extract can be used as a poultice and applied to a sore on the skin. It helps fight bacterial infections. *Ragwort* can be used as a dressing to relieve inflammation. Caution: *Ragwort* is not recommended for ingestion. The rootstock of the *pink lady's slipper* can be steeped with

"A few of these plants may be enjoyed as a tea, daily, for the benefit of your health. You can use two or three at a time, mixing equal parts of the roots and/or leaves thoroughly. Use one heaping teaspoon per one cup of boiling water. Read their descriptions and decide which is best for you."

"Bayberry is great for the immune system. It cleanses the liver, can be used as a mouthwash for sore throats, and relieves symptoms due to the menstruation cycle."

"Golden Seal contains anti – inflammatory and laxative properties. It also aids in digestion."

"Lady's Slipper helps relieve pain due to nerves and muscle spasms. It's a natural tonic; it soothes and relaxes the mind, and helps ease anxiety."

Flo

bastard toadflax (an herbaceous parasite) and the juice can be dabbed on an open sore. *Bogbean* leaves can be used as a poultice to reduce swelling. *Ground Ivy* can be steeped as a tea for the treatment of lung ulcers. A solution, also known as *Musket Shot Water,* which is made from the seeds and leaves of *bittersweet agrimony,* can be used as an herbal cure for external wounds.   Making tea from *raspberry leaves* is also good for ridding the mouth of canker sores.

Leviticus 26:16

Ague is an illness that causes fever and shivering. In this scripture the disease would affect the eyes and cause life to wane.

Eye trouble can be caused from a deranged stomach. The eyes receive their nourishment from the food taken into the stomach. Eating unhealthy foods and drinks such as: soft drinks, coffee, alcoholic beverages, fast food, sweets, etc., weakens the nerves and hinders the circulation of blood to the eyes. Poor diet contributes towards impure blood. When impure blood is carried to the eyes, it weakens them. The most important thing is to eat food that is good for the blood stream and therefore good for the body.

Treatment: To help improve ocular health it is necessary to correct the diet and give up unhealthy foods and drinks. Get plenty of sleep in a well-ventilated room. Cleanse the body with herbal enemas; blood purifying herbs, fruits, and vegetables like cucumbers, carrots, celery, and leafy greens. Take the juice of a lemon in a cup of hot water every morning before breakfast. This helps to flush the body of toxins.

There are two basic methods for treating eye problems with herbs. One method is to use an eyecup. The other method, suitable for treating both eyes at the same time, is to saturate a soft cloth with the preparation and use as a warm (or cold) press.

To treat inflammation of the eye, steep one teaspoon of *red raspberry leaves* and one teaspoon of *witch hazel leaves* in a cup of boiling water, then strain. Soak a soft cloth with the tea and apply it as a warm press over the eyes. Cold *slippery elm* poultice applied to the eyes will relieve inflammation as well. An excellent eyewash for every day use is one teaspoon of *golden seal* to one level teaspoon of boric acid dissolved in a pint of boiling water, and shaken well. After the solution settles, you can use it as eyewash. Caution: Boric acid solutions should not be used on infants.

II King 4: 18 – 20

Sunstroke or heatstroke is caused by direct overexposure to the sun. Long exposure in high temperatures, laboring in extreme heat, or lying in the sun too long can lead to sunstroke, or failure of the body's natural mechanism for regulating body heat. Sunstroke can be a serious threat to the life of an individual when treatment is delayed. Symptoms of heatstroke include: headache, dizziness, nausea, collapse, little or no sweating, flush, dry skin, a racing pulse, fast breathing, and a fever of 106 degrees or more.

Treatment: If the fever is high it must be brought down quickly to avoid shock, convulsions, delirium, coma, and/or death. Call a physician or ambulance at once. Meanwhile, place the person in a tub of ice water and rub the skin until the temperature falls. Take the temperature, by rectum, every ten minutes until 102 degrees is reached, then stop cooling. If the temperature continues to drop then the person must be kept warm. Massage the body to prevent the blood vessels from constricting. If the temperature goes up again, return the person to the tub of cold water. With prompt and correct treatment, followed by several days of care, total recovery can be expected.

Heat exhaustion, although similar to sunstroke in producing dizziness and headache, is a relatively minor disorder and is unlike sunstroke in other ways. Heat exhaustion may follow long exposure to heat or too much activity under the hot sun. The skin is clammy and cold instead of flushed and hot, as in sunstroke. Sweating is profuse instead of absent, the pulse rate is not high, nor is there a significant fever. Other symptoms of heat exhaustion may include weakness and dimming or blurring of vision. To treat heat exhaustion lye down in a cool place with the head lower than the rest of the body. Slowly sip water and take salt tablets to replenish lost fluids and salt.

II King 20:7

An **abscess** is a boil. Boils and carbuncles are generally caused by infection in a hair follicle.

Treatment: A poultice made of ground *flaxseed*, *peach tree leaves*, and *catnip leaves* (or *roasted onions*) and applied hot will draw the infection to a pit. *Yarrow leaves*, powdered *slippery elm* (or *wheat bran*), *plantain leaves*, and lard boiled and applied while warm is also a good alternative. Soaking the boil in hot Epsom salt water will also aid in relieving a person of an abscess.

Burdock tea, *gentian root* tea, *wild cherry bark* tea, *red clover* tea, *yellow dock root* tea, *sarsaparilla* or *sassafras* tea are all natural blood purifiers. Drinking tea that cleans the blood will help keep one free of boils and carbuncles.

Matthew 12:10 – 13

Atrophy is when body tissue or organs begin to waste away.

Treatment: According to important studies, the vitamin which one can most depend upon to help prevent the hallmarks of old age, loss of teeth, shrinking in stature, wrinkling of the skin, and other symptoms is said to be vitamin C. While vitamin E is considered one of the best for keeping the body in good shape, it is now known that vitamin C provides tremendous support for the body. This vitamin helps the body resist and recover from destructive attacks from sickness and disease. It is the prerequisite for the formation of collagen, an essential protein in teeth, bone cartilage, connective tissue, and skin. The need for regenerating collagen is the prime reason that vitamin C requirements increase with age. An anti-wrinkle lotion can be made with a half-ounce of glycerin, half-ounce of rosewater, half-ounce of *witch hazel*, and three tablespoons of honey. Massaging warm *olive oil* into the forehead is said to help overcome wrinkles. You may also add a few drops of *Balm of Gilead* (*Cottonwood oil*) to *barley* water and use to help reduce the appearance of wrinkles as well.

Exodus 9:10

Blains are a violent ulcerous inflammation; it's a local bodily response to injury in which an affected area becomes, red, hot, painful and filled with blood, such as cancer.

Cancer is increasing at an alarming rate, and yet can be prevented. Through chronic autointoxication, constipation, and inactivity of all the organs of elimination, such as: lungs, kidneys, skin, and bowels, the system becomes poisoned, and the poisons accumulate around the weakest organs or where a blow, fall, or bruise has injured the body. The poisoning of the body has been caused by the use of improper foods, as well as the use of caffeinated tea, coffee, coca cola, liquor of all kinds, tobacco in all forms, etc.

Among the improper foods are meat, especially pork, cane sugar, and cane sugar products; white flour products, white rice, and all denatured foods, which cause waste matter in the system. Cancer would be rare if no devitalized foods and meats were eaten. Consuming life-giving

> *"In II Sam. 24: 15 – 25 we read about a pestilence or plague the Lord sent upon the Israelites. A plague is considered to be a severe kind of typhus accompanied by buboes (tumors). There are many kinds of tumors. They are named according to the tissues involved, such as glandular, muscular, fibrous, fatty, and there are also cancerous tumors. Any one of these tumors may enlarge rapidly and become ulcerated."*
>
> *Flo*

properties keep the blood stream pure, and cancer will not develop where there is a pure blood stream.

Treatment: The first step is to cleanse the blood stream thoroughly relieving constipation, and making all the organs of elimination active. Keep the skin, lungs, liver, kidneys, and bowels active. For constipation, take an herbal laxative, use high enemas to cleanse and cure the colon of any bad condition. It may be necessary to take a fruit diet of oranges, grapefruit, lemons, apples, cranberries, unsweetened blueberries, red raspberries, cherries, peaches, pears, ripe strawberries, avocados, pineapples, and tomatoes. All fruit should be well ripened on the tree or vine to be fully beneficial.

Tomatoes should be eaten apart from other foods. Make a meal of them. For the first ten days (or a longer or shorter period depending upon the condition of the person) it is advisable to take nothing but unsweetened fruit juices, preferably orange, grapefruit, pineapple, lemon, or grape. Do not mix the juices but take different ones at different times. Vegetable juices made with celery, cucumbers, parsley, lettuce, and carrots are very useful. Carrot juice is especially valuable. Carrots contain powerful antioxidants, alpha carotene, and beta-carotene, which are cancer preventatives.

Get plenty of fresh air and exercise outdoors in the sunshine, if possible, to cleanse the lungs and increase circulation. If one is unable to be outdoors, find a sunshiny and well-ventilated room to deep breath or exercise in. Thorough messaging is very necessary in the treatment of cancer to assist in the elimination of poisons from the body.

One of the great causes of cancer is the food we eat. Statistics show that one of the top ten cancers among men and women are in the colon and rectum. I believe this is caused directly by improper foods and eating habits. A faulty diet irritates the stomach and can develop ulcers in the digestive system, which, if not cured, develops into cancer. I believe this is what happens without the person ever realizing what is taking place inside of them, until the cancer has developed.

Violet leaves (or you may use the whole plant) have been known to cure cancer when the diet and other habits were corrected. Make a tea of the leaves by using   one-half ounce of the leaves to a pint of boiling water. Steep one-half an hour and drink a cupful every two hours. If possible, dip a piece of cloth into some of this tea and apply warm over the affected part and leave on until dry. A poultice is made of fresh *violet* leaves chopped and steeped in boiling water for thirty minutes. Then add linseed meal to thicken the solution. As an enema use one-half ounce of the solution to a pint of water and inject night and morning. Using *bittersweet agrimony* and *ground ivy* are also excellent; they heal by drying up the cancer.

Here is a list of herbs, that can be taken as a tea, to help ward off cancer: *red clover blossoms, burdock root, yellow dock root, blue violet (the whole plant), golden seal root, gum myrrh, Echinacea, aloes, blue flag, gravel root, blood root, dandelion root, African cayenne, chickweed, rock rose, agrimony, and Oregon grape. Red Clover* tea helped my father-in-law who had stage-three cancer. He was only given a year to live but he lived beyond that.

Deuteronomy 28:22

Consumption was a plague that affected the land. It is a sickness that causes the body to waste away, such as tuberculosis, which was then called consumption. Let's use tuberculosis as the subject for consumption.

Tuberculosis may affect, not only the lungs, but also other parts of the body such as: the liver, spleen, intestines, spine, and bones. Intemperance in eating, drinking, dressing, exposure to cold, impure air, lack of proper exercise, and improper breathing can pave the way for tuberculosis to develop. Loss of sleep, malnourishment, being overworked, a sedentary life, and an unbalanced diet can be contributing factors as well. Contaminated milk, use of tobacco in any form, liquor of all kinds, caffeinated tea, coffee, and other harmful drinks can also be active causes. Persons with feeble constitutions are those mostly affected with tuberculosis.

Usually slow in developing, a habitual cough, gradually becoming severe, causing vomiting and profuse expectoration, the person becomes extremely weak, is subject to night sweats and bleeding from the lungs.

Treatment: A moderate temperature should be maintained at all times, never having it excessively warm and always having good ventilation. Avoid becoming chilled. The person's room should be sunny, airy, and dry. Get plenty of outdoor exercise and stay outdoors as much as possible.

Steep one teaspoon of powdered *golden seal* and one teaspoon of *lobelia* in a pint of boiling water for one half hour. Take a swallow every hour. Mix two tablespoons of powdered *bugleweed* with a pinch of *cayenne* and use a level teaspoon of this mixture to a cup of boiling water. Take a swallow of this every two hours. A cupful of this tea is also useful to check bleeding from the lungs. Powdered *bayberry bark* or *shepherd's purse* is also very good to check hemorrhage of the lungs. Use half a teaspoon to a cup of boiling water, let steep, strain, and drink cold.

Drink at least on quart of *slippery elm* tea daily, drinking one cup an hour before each meal and one at bedtime. It will strengthen, heal, and nourish. If the digestion is not good, take one-fourth teaspoon of powdered *golden seal* in a glass of water an hour before each meal.

A nourishing diet is necessary. Soybean milk can be taken freely. Soybean milk with whole-wheat flakes is very nourishing. Other good foods to use in the diet are: very ripe bananas, oatmeal with malt honey, and whole wheat, or soybean bread, zwieback, potassium broth, tender fresh peas, steamed figs, dates, graham crackers, all kinds of vegetables (seasoned with soybean milk or soybean butter), natural brown rice, and baked Irish potatoes.

Deep breathing and plenty of fresh air are necessary in connection with gentle exercise. Sunbaths are excellent; expose the entire body. Take sweat baths to open the pores while drinking two or three cups of tea, made from *pleurisy root*, while in the tub.

All sputa and discharges of the person suffering from tuberculosis or consumption should be burned or buried.

Matthew 9:27

Blindness is when one cannot see.

In a sense, the increase in blindness, in recent years, is a result of the great strides taken by the medical field. For example, blindness as a result of diabetes is on the rise, largely because the life span of most diabetics can now be prolonged by use of medicine. Before the discovery of insulin, most victims of diabetes died before the disease could cause blindness. Similarly, failing eyesight, caused by degeneration of the arteries, is increasing because our higher health standards mean that many people live to the age when they are susceptible to this disease. A major cause of blindness today is cataract, a clouding of the eye lens. The second major cause is chronic glaucoma, an increase in fluid pressure inside the eyeball. This pressure damages the optic nerve. Trachoma, a major viral infection of the eyes, was once a major cause of blindness in the United States and still is in many other countries.

Treatment: Natural antibiotics can help halt the disease. *Ginkgo* and *bilberry* are two herbs that help increase circulation around the eyes. Eating a diet high in omega – 3 and antioxidants will help slow the progression of failing eyesight. Once again, carrots should be included in the diet regularly as it provides beta-carotene, another antioxidant that defends against blindness.

Mark 7:32

Deafness is when one is wholly or partly unable hear, or unwilling to hear.

Deafness caused by cholesterol deposits in the arteries of the ears is said to clean up when the blood cholesterol is kept consistently low. Persons who are hard of hearing have particularly low blood iodine and a lack of iodine during pregnancy can cause deafness in an infant.

Treatment: The herbs and plants to take, as a tea, for deafness are: *chickweed*, *origanum*, *marjoram*, *angelica*, oil of *wintergreen*, oil of *sassafras*, tincture of *myrrh*, and tincture of *lobelia*.

Psalm 102:23

Debility is when a person is in a weak or infirmed state.

If the individual cannot burn off the carbon in the body properly the person will feel weak most of the time. The greater the consumption of carbon: the greater the need for oxygen. Small amounts of oxygen and larger amounts of carbon result in weak flabby muscles.

Treatment: Native Americans used *golden seal root* tea for indigestion, low fevers, and for general weakness. It was also used as a wash for inflammation of the eye.

Luke 14:2 – 4

Dropsy is an abnormal accumulation of watery fluid in the bodily tissue or in any of the cavities of the body. It is more so known, today, as Edema, and may be due to disease of the heart, lungs, liver, kidney, or peritoneum. Anything that will cause the blood to become poisoned or the red corpuscles to die may result in dropsy. Edema may also occur as the result of heart or liver failure.

Treatment: Generally, a complete change should be made in the diet, leaving off all alcoholic drinks, cocoa, chocolate, caffeinated tea, coffee, coca cola, and all other soft drinks. There should be no indulgence in flesh food, pies, cakes, or rich pastries. All foods should be eaten as dry as possible, thereby causing the person to chew his food thoroughly. No fluid should be taken with meals; water can be consumed one hour after meals. Do not use any salt. Fruits or tomatoes should compose a large part of the diet. One vegetable meal a day (preferably at noon) should compose the diet of all persons. Don't eat fruit and vegetables at the same mealtime.

Sprouted lentils and sprouted soybeans are very good. Eat freely of vegetables such as: eggplant, young beets, parsley, celery, okra, kale, asparagus, collard greens, mustard greens, lettuce, spinach, parsnip onions, cucumbers, watercress, pumpkin, potatoes, peas, yellow corn, Swiss chard, cauliflower, endive, fresh beans, and peas.

Drinking plenty of herbal teas, *red raspberry* or *pleurisy root* will produce perspiration. If the herb is in a powdered form, take a half teaspoonful to one cup of boiling water. Let it steep thirty minutes and drink. The powder may also be taken in capsules four to six times a day. An excellent herb combination for this purpose is one half teaspoonful (each) of *wild yam* and *black cohosh*, with a pinch of *cayenne pepper*, to a cup of water.

Keep the bowels active, so that they move at least three times a day, by using the herbal laxatives as given in this book. A tea made of the following may be taken freely, as much as four to six cups a day with benefit: *Wild carrot* (blossoms or seeds ground), *dandelion root, yarrow, burdock root, queen of the meadow, dwarf elder,* and *broom.* This may be mixed with equal parts, using one teaspoon to a cup of boiling water, and steeping twenty or thirty minutes.

Matthew 9:32 – 33

Dumbness is when one is lacking the normal power of speech or is not willing to speak. There is no herb for this sickness, but a holy ghost filled person, *anointed to pray and lay hands on the individual,* can call out the dumb demon.

Acts 28:8

Dysentery is a disease characterized by severe diarrhea with passage of mucus and blood from the bowels.

Inflammation of the rectum and large intestines can be caused by inadequate food and improper diet, drinking with meals, overeating, wrong combinations, stimulating foods and liquors, the use of tobacco, caffeinated tea and coffee, and drinking impure water. Unhygienic environments, eating decomposed foods, fruits, or vegetables, and eating foods that have been stored in pantries that are not well ventilated can also be contributing factors. Habitual constipation will inflame the rectum as well.

Treatment: First, give a high enema using either: *white oak bark*, *bayberry bark*, or *wild alum root* tea. Give enemas as hot as can be tolerated, between 102 and 108 degrees Fahrenheit. It may be hard to retain the tea at a hot temperature but it will give great relief. In severe cases it may be given a little warmer. Give hot fomentation to the abdomen and spine continuing for a half an hour, and if the case is severe give three or four times a day. These are indispensable. The liniment to use for the abdomen and spine is two ounces of powdered *myrrh*, one ounce powdered *golden seal*, one half-ounce *cayenne pepper*, and one quart rubbing alcohol (70%). Mix together and let stand seven days; shake well every day. Pour the mixture into corked bottles for storage. If you do not have *golden seal* then make the mixture without it.

I Samuel 5:9

Emerods or hemorrhoids are known as piles or bleeding piles when they become swollen, inflamed, or irritated.

A poor diet, overeating, intoxicating liquors, tobacco, spices of various kinds, white bread, sugar, fried foods, and all acid forming foods which cause fermentation can irritate hemorrhoids. This devitalized diet causes constipation, clogs the liver, causes an impure blood stream, and irritates the stomach and intestines. Taking ordinary purgatives that are on the market are also a cause, as they irritate the membranous lining of the bowel and intestines.

Treatment: First, use a high hot enema, temperature from 102 to 108 degrees Fahrenheit. Use either: *white oak bark*, *bayberry bark*, or *wild alum root* tea. This will cleanse the entire length of the colon. Make a strong tea of *witch hazel bark* with one teaspoon of *yellow dock root*. If you do not have the other herbs, you may use just the *witch hazel bark* or *catnip* to a cup of boiling water and steep for twenty minutes. If the trouble is external, dip a small piece of cotton in this tea and bathe the affected area. If they are internal, get a baby syringe and inject two tablespoons at a time. You will find that this will give relief in no time.

When taking herbal enemas you will find that it is less painful and the piles will go back inside easier if you take the knee-chest position, as this causes the intestines to drop forward. Also, remember to consult a physician or holistic doctor before starting an enema.

All heavy and stimulating foods should be avoided. Foods to be avoided include: tobacco, caffeinated tea, coffee, vinegar, alcoholic beverages, and fatty meats of all kinds. The diet should be simple and light. Potassium broth is very excellent. Soybean milk, soybean zwieback, thoroughly ripe bananas, and vegetable broth of any kind are great foods to consume. Going on a fruit diet for a few days is also a helpful measure.

Matthew 4:24

Epilepsy is a disorder marked by disturbed electrical rhythms of the central nervous system, and characterized by convulsive attacks and loss of consciousness.

A poor diet can be a major cause. A poor diet will cause the stoppage of bowels and affect the sympathetic nerves, which in turn will affect the cerebra-spinal nerves. This condition calls all the blood away from the head, which at times almost stops the heart, and causes the face to become very pale, or purple, and the body to limp. It is often caused from trouble in the bowels and intestines or can be caused by falls, blows, fractures, and other injuries. There are also cases where the epilepsy is caused by worms, also known as a parasitic infection.

Treatment: Have some antispasmodic tincture on hand and put eight to fifteen drops in one half of a glass of water. If the person cannot drink, put a few drops on the tongue. This will check the fit at once. Give a high enema of *catnip* tea immediately to relieve and cleanse the bowels thoroughly.

When the attack first comes on, or during the duration of the fit, have the person lie down and have plenty of fresh air in the room. When and if possible give the antispasmodic tincture before the attack.

To make a tea that is excellent for use in epilepsy, mix equal parts of the following herbs: *black cohosh*, *valerian*, *lady's slipper*, and *skullcap*. Steep a heaping teaspoon of this mixture in a cup of boiling water for thirty minutes. Have the person drink two or three cups of this, just as warm as possible, when or if he or she feels the attack coming on. This tea should be continued after the attack as well. If the person complains of pain in the bowels, apply liniment as given in this book. Rub it freely and thoroughly. Caution: Only a physician or health care professional can diagnose an epileptic seizure or seizure of any type. Call a paramedic, physician, or other health care professional in any matter where there is a seizure involved.

Matthew 8:14

A **fever** occurs when the body's temperature rises above normal.

The body is filled with waste matter and the fever is nature's process of burning up impurities.

Treatment: Take an emetic to cleanse the stomach. Should the temperature be too high, and the person too ill for this, give a cup of *golden seal* and *myrrh.* This will kill the poison in the stomach. To make a pint of this tea, steep a heaping teaspoon of *golden seal* and one half of a teaspoon of *myrrh* in a pint of boiling water for twenty minutes. After taking the first cupful, take a tablespoonful every hour thereafter. More can be taken with benefit.

Cool water enemas will bring down the temperature rapidly. Have the water slightly below body temperature. An herb enema is more effective, however Castile or ivory soap may be used; have the water slightly sudsy. It is the removal of the poisons from the system that brings the temperature down. Remove the person's clothes and put him or her between cotton blankets. Sponge off all over with tepid water, beginning with the face, sponge downward over the entire body, sponging well around the head and the back of the neck. Sponge the feet thoroughly, leaving the sole moist. Do this every five minutes in high fevers. Give sips of cold water every five minutes. In case the person becomes too chilly, stop the bath, cover well, and place hot water bottles or hot fomentations over the stomach. This will usually stop the chill. If it does not, apply hot fomentations to the spine or give a hot footbath. A hot drink should also check the chill at once.

The bowels should be kept open with an herbal laxative. Sometimes lemon juice alone will break the fever if it is a low fever. *Slippery elm* tea is good in all feverish cases. It is also a powerful cleanser, soothing to the stomach and intestinal tract.

Anyone of the following herbs are useful in fevers: *yarrow, catnip, peppermint, red sage, valerian,* and *chamomile.* Make a tea and drink copiously until the fever abates. *Red raspberry leaf* tea is excellent for reducing fever in children.

Deuteronomy 28:22

Inflammation is a local bodily response to trauma in which the affected area becomes red, hot, painful, and filled with blood.

Treatment: The *chamomile* flowers can be made into a rubbing oil for swellings, calloused skin, and painful joints. *Chamomile* tea is good for using as a wash on open sores and wombs. It can also be taken for colic fever, dyspepsia, flatulence, and restlessness in children.

German chamomile tea tends to reduce inflammation. It can also be used as a wash or compress for skin problems and inflammation, including inflammation of mucus tissue. *German chamomile* tea is also valuable in many nervous conditions, insomnia, neuralgia, lumbago, rheumatic problems, and rashes. It can facilitate bowel movements without acting directly as a purgative. Keeping a mouthful of the tea in the mouth for a time will temporarily relieve toothache. To help asthma in children or to relieve the symptoms of a cold, try a vapor bathe of the tea. *German chamomile* can also be used as a relaxing, antispasmodic, anodyne bath additive. Use it for a sitz bath to help hemorrhoids, or as a foot or hand bath for sweaty feet and hands. The flowers can also be made into salve for applying on hemorrhoids and wounds.

Daniel 4:33 – 34

Insanity is the senseless conduct or extreme unsoundness or derangement of the mind, also considered a mental illness or disorder.

Treatment: The *holy thistle* plant is powerful in the purification and circulation of the blood. It is very effective for dropsy, strengthens the heart, and is good for the liver, lungs, and kidneys. It is soothing to the brain, strengthens the memory, clears the system of bad humors, and is effective for insanity. It is a good tonic for girls entering womanhood. It is claimed that the warm tea is good for nursing mothers producing a free supply of milk.

Deuteronomy 28:27

An **itch** is an uneasy and irritating sensation in the skin.

There are various kinds of itches: seven-year itch, Barber's itch, and bricklayer's itch among others. A very small insect called an "itch mite" caused the itch that went by the name of seven-year itch for a great many years. They bore beneath the skin where it is thin or warm and moist. This is usually between the fingers, wrists, forearm, etc. In children, they attack the feet, hands, and buttocks, the itching being greater at night when the body is warm. Scratching the irritation causes pimples and scabs. The following treatment is helpful in the case of chiggers or anything of that nature.

Treatment: Before each application of the following, thoroughly wash the affected parts with tar soap. All clothing must be washed with boiling water. When they cannot be washed or boiled, press with a hot iron to destroy any insects that may be on them.

Take one tablespoonful each of the following; *burdock root, yellow dock root,* and *yarrow,* steep in a pint of boiling water for a half an hour. Strain through a cloth and put in a granite-cooking pan (do not use aluminum), add one pound of cocoa fat, or Crisco. Boil this slowly, stirring frequently, until it has boiled down to the consistency of a salve. This is an excellent salve for an itch or eczema of any kind. If you do not wish to make the salve, bathe the affected parts with tea as directed above.

II Kings 5:1

Leprosy is a chronic bacterial disease that progresses slowly. Spreading and swelling is accompanied by loss of sensation, wasting, and deformities.

Leprosy is a very ancient disease, more common in the tropics and along the seashores where people live largely upon fish and meats, and eat very few fruits and vegetables. The skin becomes spotted and there is a break out which continues to grow and become ulcerated and decayed, even the bones decay. There is loss of feeling in the affected parts; the fingers and toes drop off from decomposition.

Treatment: Fresh air and a nourishing diet are essential. Fish and meats of all kinds are strictly forbidden. Eat plenty of fresh fruits.

An excellent herbal composition for leprosy is one heaping teaspoon of *red clover* blossoms, one teaspoon of *yellow dock root*, one teaspoon of *calamus*, one teaspoon of *burdock*, and one-half teaspoon of *mandrake*. Mix it together and use a heaping teaspoonful to a cup of boiling water. Drink four cups a day, one hour before each meal, and one hot cup before retiring.

Matthew 4:24

Palsy is the loss of sensation or motion in any part of the body.

Palsy is a nervous physical condition due to fatigue, or the use of caffeinated tea, coffee, liquor, and stimulating foods. All refined food products like white flour and cane sugar can be contributing factors, as they lack properties that sustain and strengthen the nerves. Collapse in one form or another is always the result of living on a diet composed mainly of such foods.

Caffeinated tea, coffee, liquor and all stimulating foods must not be used if a person wants to be cured. All the good food that may be eaten cannot do the body any good until one has eliminated and cleansed the body of excess acids and mucous. The intestines retain these poisons and they are one of the main causes of the disease and old age. To eliminate these unnatural, unhealthful conditions and make it possible for food to be assimilated and absorbed by the system, the body must be flushed and cleansed. Eating healthy foods will bring about natural rejuvenation by constantly supplying the blood stream with natural elements, of which they are originally composed, as found in natural foods, eaten raw or cooked so as not to destroy their mineral or life giving properties. You will be feeding the entire body.

Treatment: Hot and cold applications to the affected parts with vigorous massaging afterwards are very beneficial; this increases circulation. A warm bath and a salt glow rub can also be given with good results. The pores of the skin must be open and a good circulation started. Take laxative herbs enough, so you will have three or four good bowel movements a day.

Steep one tablespoon of *prickly ash bark* or berries, a pinch of *cayenne*, and one teaspoon of *lobelia* in a pint of boiling water. Take a tablespoon every two hours.

GAS IN THE STOMACH AND BOWELS

Gas in the stomach and bowels is the result of a problem with digestion. The food remains in the stomach too long and becomes fermented and sour. A small measure of wrong food combinations will cause gas in the stomach and bowels. Drinking with meals causes sour stomach and fermentation, as does hasty eating and poor mastication.

Treatment: *Peppermint* and *spearmint* tea are good for overcoming gas in the stomach. Equal parts of *calamus root*, valerian, with *peppermint* or *spearmint*, granulated, should be taken. Mix together, and use a teaspoon to a cup of boiling water, steep, strain, and drink one-half cupful an hour before meals, and another half cupful after meals. The above herbs can be used in powdered form as well as capsules, if desired.

To strengthen the stomach and cleanse it so that this condition will be overcome, take one-fourth a teaspoon of powdered *golden seal* in one half a glass of warm water an hour before each meal. If you prefer, you may take it as follows: one heaping teaspoonful *golden seal* and one-fourth teaspoon of *myrrh* to a pint of boiling water, steep and take a swallow just

a few minutes before eating.

WOMB TROUBLE

One of the most common causes of vaginal discharge, inflammation, itching, and perhaps pain during and after intercourse is a parasitic infection known as trichomoniasis. Itching around the genitals has improved tremendously when women have been given as little as six milligrams of vitamin B2 daily. A rash or dermatitis in the vagina, accompanied by swelling, itching, and even bleeding, has cleared up when vitamin B2, or B6, or both have been taken. Inflammation and itching of the vagina has also been helped by vitamin E. Leukorrhea and inflammation have disappeared after vitamin A was given.

Treatment: An extremely good treatment for female troubles is made up of the following: a thick paste made of powdered *slippery elm* and pure cold water. Shape into pieces about one inch long and one inch thick. Place in warm water for a few minutes. These are called vaginal suppositories. Insert three followed by a tampon afterwards. Let it remain two days.

Remove the tampon and give a douche, which will remove the slippery elm. (In case of congestion it is best to douche using one gallon of water as warm as possible.) This will help in treating cancer and tumors of the womb, growths in the female organs, fallen womb, leukorrhea, or inflammation and congestion of any part of the vagina or womb. *Slippery elm* will roll up the mucous material that's troubling the person and pass it down through the intestines. It cleans, heals, and strengthens.

HEBREWS IN THE LAND OF MILK & HONEY

How did the people of the Holy Land live in the days of Abraham, Moses, Solomon, Isaiah, Ruth, and Esther? What types of clothing did they wear? What did they use for food? How did they heal their ailments? An amazing number of clues can be found in a study of plants that are mentioned in the Bible. Even modern researchers have identified many Old Testament plants.

The river Jordan flows into the Dead Sea at about 400+ meters below sea level, while at the northern end of the Jordan Valley the heights of Mt. Hermon and Mt. Lebanon are capped with snow for most of the year. Extending from the borders of the Mediterranean to the foothills of the mountains are three valleys, the Plain of Sharon, the Plain of Esdraelon (Jezreel Valley), and the valley of Elah. These alone are rich subtropical areas of agriculture, the "Land of Milk and Honey."

In early biblical times, life was seminomadic, half way between a desert Bedouin and a settled farmer. We read of Isaac sowing, Joseph binding sheaves, and Reuben in the harvest field. The semi nomads gathered olives, dates, walnuts, pistachios, and figs. When they began to form villages and towns, they grew barley, wheat, spelt, millet sorghum, flax, grapes, apricots, various vegetables, and herbs. Bread was baked daily and sometimes olive oil was added to the dough. Wafers were baked and flavored with honey and cakes were sprinkled with aromatic herbs. Since water was scarce, goats and sheep provided milk for drinking and making cheese and butter.

In addition to bread and milk, the ordinary diet consisted mainly of vegetables such as: cucumbers, broad beans, leeks, onions, and garlic. There were soups of lentils and beans; on certain occasions meats were eaten, flavored and preserved by a variety of spices. Standard foods for soldiers, travelers, and field workers were raisins and parched grain. For dessert, there were fruit, fresh and dried figs, grapes, apricots, melons, pomegranates, pistachios, almonds, and walnuts were relished. Wine was universal; other alcoholic beverages were made from dates and pomegranates. Pomegranates also provided the base for several non-alcoholic drinks, as did licorice root.

During their wandering in the wilderness, the Israelites probably lived largely on manna, which even today, is a favorite confection in many eastern lands. According to the Bible manna is from Heaven, however, in nature manna has various identifications. It has also been identified as a sap or gum exuded from a variety of plants, including alhagi (Sinai manna), tamarisk flowering ash, and lecanora lichen. Manna has also been considered to be the end result of the scale insects, after they suck up sap from plants, and secrete drops of fluid that dry into sticky sweet solids on the body of the host plant.

Fabrics of all kinds were also made from plants. While some sackcloth was woven from goat hair, other varieties were made from coarse flax, papyrus, and even almond stalks. Ordinary linen was used for towels, lamp wicks, nets, sails, and flags. Fine linen made turbans, veils, undergarments, as well as raiment for royalty and priests. Wool was used to make clothing exclusively for the wealthy. While cotton and silk were used, they were entirely imported. Cotton came from Egypt and India; silk was brought from China.

For cooking of all kinds, from drugs and cosmetics to perfumes and dyes, the people turned to herbs and trees. For example, aromatic coriander leaves flavored soups and wines, while coriander seeds made condiments and medicines. The pistils of the saffron crocus were used for seasoning, food coloring, and were also used on perfumes, and as an important yellow dye. Marjoram was probably the biblical "hyssop" which served for purification and in cleansing lepers. Perfumery was of particular importance in biblical times; both for daily use and for ritual functions, and in many cases the same plants were employed in perfumes and medicines. For instance, the rare and costly gum from the Balm of Gilead, a small evergreen tree, was ingredient to both. Wormwood, a name given to several woody plants with a strong aromatic odor, was also used in medicine and perfumery. The "aloes" of the Old Testament were not true aloes as they are thought to be Eaglewood (Agarwood).

Naturally, the Hebrews included local plant product in the incense and anointing oils used for religious ceremonies. During the Feast of Tabernacles, myrtle and willow branches were braided with palm fronds to form sacra luau, which was held in the right hand during the ritual. At the same time, a citron (the fruit of a goodly tree), also known as "Ethrogh", ceremonially was held in the left hand.

The "cassia" of the Bible refers to two different plants. In Exodus, Proverbs, and Psalms it refers to the cassia bark (cinnamon), a common spice and perfume. The ripe fruits of the tree yield oil of cinnamon, one of the ingredients in the holy oil. Officiating priests in the Tabernacle were anointed with this oil. Another cassia is the Indian Orris, a thistle-life plant that was widely used as a Temple fragrance and incense; frankincense was also used. It often came from the tree Boswellia Carteri; its bitter and much sought after gum was used in the sacrificial services of the Tabernacle and the Temple.

Myrrh is a gum from Cistus Illosus, a thorny shrub or small tree, native to East Africa, whose wood and bark are strongly scented. It was used in embalming, perfumery, and incense. It was also mixed with aloe, cassia, cinnamon, and olive. Myrrh was an almost indispensable ingredient in holy oil.

Another oil yielding plant was the gourd mentioned in Jonah 4:6, which has been identified as Palma Christi, the common castor oil plant. The oil, obtained from the large seeds, was used extensively in ceremonies, as was the perfumed gum "stacte", mentioned in Exodus. Stacte was produced from the sweet Storax, a small tree with beautiful aromatic flowers.

The Bay tree or Bay Laurel, sometimes-called Sweet Bay, was an evergreen that also figured in religious ceremonies. Its aromatic leaves flavored food; the roots and bark supplied medicine. It was a mark of triumph, adorning the brows of the priests, poets, and victors. David used the Laurel as a symbol of prosperity.

References to flowers abound in the scriptures. Unfortunately, many are not mentioned by name and some of the names that are given are so vague. Translators and botanists agree that the Hebrew (Shushan) word once translated as "lily" or "lilies of the field", refers to the anemone or windflower. The "lily of the valley", on the other hand is believed to be the Hyacinth, whose blue blossoms brighten both fields and rocky places. Another "lily" is the Iris, or Yellow Flag, that grows in shallow waters on the margins of ponds and streams, and sometimes in extensive masses.

The "Rose" of the Bible is thought to be the Narcissus in some passages, and Oleander in others. The "Rose of Sharon" refers to the tulip. "Doves Dung" is the Star of Bethlehem, a spring flowering plant whose bulbs served as food during times of drought and starvation. "Tirzah", in the Song of Solomon 6:4, is acknowledged to be the Crocus.

The grapevine is the first cultivated plant mentioned in the Bible. There are more references to "vine growing" and "wine" than to any other plant or product. Grapes supplied fresh fruit, raisins, a sweet syrup known as "dibs" and vinegar, as well as alcoholic beverage. There are many laws in the Old Testament on the selection, planting, care, harvesting, pressing, storing, and tithing of vines, grapes, and wine.

Trees, many of which were venerated as sacred, played important roles in the lives of people in the Holy Land. There is a great deal of controversy over hundreds of tree references in the Bible, as well as the identity of the evergreens, especially fir, pine, cypress, juniper, and cedar.

The cedar of Lebanon is one of the most sacred of Biblical trees. Chief among the evergreens, it was known as the "Prince of Trees", a symbol of grandeur, might, majesty, and dignity. Many Lebanon cedars are over 2,000 years old. Their wood is so rot resistant that they were cut in great quantities to construct Solomon's "House of Cedar" and the Temple.

The great cypress forests of the biblical days were called gopher wood groves because of their durability; cypress was used to build idols and ships. Cypress may have also furnished Noah with wood from which he constructed the ark.

The very word "Palestine" means "land of palms". All manner of foods: beverages, confections, ornaments, fuel, household utensils, clothing, footwear, and cordage were supplied by flowers, fruits, seeds, fronds, and the trunk of the palm. For the Hebrews, the palm was a token of triumph, carried in processions. Indeed, the Israelites' Palm Festival preceded today's Christian Palm Sunday.

As important as the palm was, both economically and religiously, the olive tree symbolized peace. Its gnarled trunk and spreading silver green foliage remain characteristic features of the Mediterranean landscape. Moses called the land of Canaan a "land of olive oil". In addition to food, the olive supplied illuminating oil and was used in soaps, cosmetics, and medicine. It was a constituent of the holy oil that was used for anointing royalty and for Temple ceremonies. Its beautiful hardwood decorated the doors of the Temple.

The almond is the first tree to flower the Holy Land and is in full bloom in January. "Shaked", the Hebrew word for almond, means "hasty awakening". This dramatized in the story of Aaron's rod, which in a single day burst into bloom and yielded almonds as a sign of the fulfillment of God's promise. Oil, ointments, and cosmetics were made from the nut, as was a favorite food flavoring.

Of all the tree fruits, the acorn may have been the first gathered by man. Forest of various species of oaks once covered hills and mountains of the Holy Land, and many of the events of Hebrew legend and history occurred beneath the oak trees. Oak worship was firmly established among the pre-Israelites of Canaan. The oak is still considered the "The King of the Forest", an emblem of majesty and strength.

The tamarisk and acacia also figure prominently in the Bible. The tamarisk, a small tree, grows in barren sandy areas where its shade is greatly appreciated. In spring it bears spikes of beautiful blossoms that envelope the whole tree. The acacias, with their aromatic long lasting wood, are among the most beautiful, fragrant, and useful of plants. Exodus 27:1 says. *"Thou shalt make an altar of shittim wood..."* and the reference is to the acacia, credited in the Bible as material for the Ark of the Covenant and the Alter of the Tabernacle. Gum Arabic, derived from these trees, was an important article of commerce; it was used in many industries. The yellow flowers were employed to the perfumery; the pods yielded feed and foods. The chips of the heartwood produced the drug catechu, and the bark was used to tan leather. One of the four "Sacred Species" of the Feast of Tabernacles is the myrtle, an aromatic evergreen shrub or tree that adorned huts or booths during this festival. Its dark glossy sweet smelling leaves, along with its white or pink perfumed flowers, and its bluish black aromatic berries were dried for condiments and perfume. In the Bible, myrtle is regarded as a symbol of divine generosity, peace, and justice.

The "sycamore", mentioned several times in the Bible, is really the sycamore fig, a tall evergreen with aromatic leaves and small spotted fruit. The common fig, one of the most important of all Bible plants, is the first tree mentioned by name, "*and they sewed fig leaves together and made themselves aprons* ", Genesis 3:7. The fig tree grows everywhere in the Middle East, among rock crevices, in old walls, and along terraces. Besides fruit for food, the small spreading tree provided welcome shade and was a symbol of tranquility. Indeed, there is scarcely a better way to end this inventory of Biblical plants than to cite I Kings 4:25, *"and Judah and Israel dwelt safely, every man under his vine and under his fig tree."*

CONCLUSION

I will conclude with a concise summary from the preamble in *Back to Eden by Jethro Kloss*.

It is with Godly fear and much humility that I undertake the task of writing this book, as I am in no sense of the word a writer. I am sending forth this book for the purpose of helping humanity and giving courage to those who may have thought their case was hopeless. My prayer is that God may make this book a blessing for many.

I wish to enlighten the general public about the untold blessings, which our Heavenly Father has provided for the entire world. It can be truly said, "My people are destroyed for lack of knowledge," Hosea 4:6. A lack of knowledge, based on the truth, is accountable for much of the sufferings and miseries that befall humanity. The advice contained in this book, if needed, will help save money, suffering, and perhaps a premature death.

From my practical experiences, I explain how to be in good health, mentally and physically. No matter how many germs get into the body, if the blood stream is clean, and the blood corpuscles are in a healthy condition, your body is in a much healthier state.

Many who violate the laws of health are ignorant of the relationship between the laws of living (eating, drinking, and moving) and good health. Until they become sick, or ill, they do not realize that violating the laws of nature and health makes the body sick. Practicing the laws of health, which include: use of pure water, fresh air, sunshine, rest, nature's remedies, herbs, etc., allows nature to restore the body to its original health. Supplying the body with these essentials all of the time keeps the body in a good condition.

There is a wonderful science in nature, in trees, herbs, roots, and flowers which man has yet to examine. God has provided a remedy for every disease that might afflict us. Satan cannot afflict anyone with any disease for which God has not provided a remedy. Our Creator foresaw the wretched condition of mankind in these days and made provision in nature for all of the troubles of man. We know this because, even for the trouble of sin, God provided a Savior.

If our scientist and medical colleges would put forth the same effort in finding the virtues in the "true remedies", as found in nature for the use of the human race, then poisonous drugs and chemicals would be eliminated and sickness would be rare indeed. If they would make use of these remedies, which God has given for the "service of man", it would bring an untold blessing to the world.

Returning to God's original plan for maintaining health, restoring the sick, miraculous truths which have been covered up by commercial graft, tradition, and neglect are being uncovered by honest men and women, and brought into the light; miraculous things are in the Bible and in nature. The Creator of this universe made man, in the beginning, out of the ground. The different properties, which are found in earth, fruits, grains, nuts, and vegetables, are also found in man. – Jethro Kloss

BIBLIOGRAPHY

Kloss, Jethro. Back To Eden. Twin Lakes, WI: Kloss Family, 1992.

Webster Intermediate Dictionary, Merriam-Webster 1972 by G.C Merriam Company.

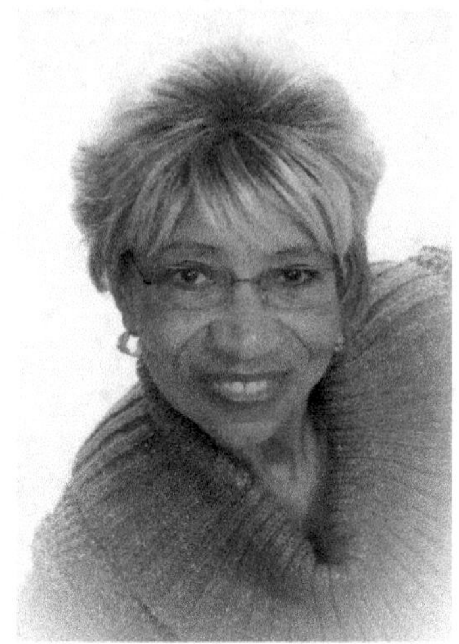

About The Author

Florastine Jethroe has dedicated herself to living for Christ Jesus. She serves in her community where she feeds the hungry, provides companionship and support for the elderly, and prayer for the infirmed. It has been her dream to share her knowledge of what God has given her about herbs and natural medicine. She credits her health to this knowledge and she honors God in it all. At seventy-four, she has five children, fifteen grandchildren, and thirteen great grandchildren.